Vegan Frozen Desserts Mastery

50 Plant-Based Ice Creams, Sorbets & Granitas

Estelle Nichols

TABLE OF CONTENTS

Copyright © 2024 by Estelle Nichols. All rights reserved. 2

TABLE OF CONTENTS 3

Part One: 5

Introduction to Frozen Vegan Desserts 5

Non-dairy ice cream 7

Fruit-Based Frozen Treats 14

Choosing an ice cream maker 16

Making, storing, and scooping homemade ice cream 18

Working without an Ice Cream Maker 20

Part 2: 22

The Recipes 22

Soymilk ice creams 24

Almond-milk ice creams 38

Coconut Milk Ice Creams 46

Sorbet and Granitas..56

Popsicles 73

Ice cream sandwiches and other frozen treats ..84

Sauces and toppings..93

Ice cream is a popular summertime pleasure. Ice cream is manufactured from milk, cream, and sugar, which give it a rich flavour and creamy texture. Making dairy-free ice cream can be simple and pleasant, despite the fact that regular ice cream typically contains milk and cream.

This collection features dairy- and egg-free vegan ice cream recipes using ingredients you may already have in your kitchen. Whether you're looking for a refreshing, sweet snack, there's something for everyone, including soy milk ice cream and fruit-infused granita.

This guide includes recipes for dairy-free whipped cream, sundae toppings, and vegan ice cream sandwiches with handmade ice cream.

Dairy-free or vegan ice creams differ from "regular" dairy ice creams because they do not contain dairy or eggs. Making vegan ice cream requires more than just substituting one ingredient. Ice cream's high fat content results in a smooth texture with few ice crystals. In certain traditional ice cream recipes, eggs are included to thicken the foundation.

A thicker base can result in a creamier finished product, but the richness of eggs might obscure flavourings. Some people prefer eggless ice cream recipes, both dairy and non-dairy, for a brighter, cleaner flavour.

Non-dairy milks contain much less fat than full-fat milk and heavy cream. Low fat ice creams include more water, resulting in more ice crystals and slower freezing compared to typical ice creams. To avoid this, use high-fat non-dairy milks like coconut milk or thicken your ice cream base with cornstarch. Adding starch, like fat, prevents ice crystals from forming, resulting in a creamier final product. Avoid using too many thickeners as they can alter the flavour of your ice cream and give it a slightly gummy feel. Typically, a modest amount is sufficient.

I avoid using non-dairy creamers and items with higher fat content compared to non-dairy milks. These products might be difficult to use and produce uneven outcomes due to extra sweeteners and chemicals. Some products are highly specialized and difficult to locate. To make these ice creams accessible to anyone, I used readily available ingredients from local grocery stores.

Ingredients: Soy milk is a soybean-derived beverage. Non-dairy milk is commonly associated with Asian cuisines. To make soy milk, dried soybeans are soaked in water, ground, then strained multiple times to remove any solvents. Soy milk typically has a similar fat percentage to low-fat milk, while non-fat options are available. Basic and flavoured versions are available, with vanilla being the most popular. Vanilla soy milk is softly sweetened and has a distinct vanilla flavour that effectively masks the earthy taste of soy milk.

I like vanilla soy milk for creating ice cream. Most vanilla soy milks perform similarly in ice cream recipes, though the amount of vanilla used may vary by type. Vanilla effectively conceals the soy flavour and complements any additional Flavors. To make soy milk ice cream creamy and prevent crystal formation in the freezer, I add thickeners to the base. **Almond milk** is a beverage prepared from almonds, comparable to soy milk. To make almond milk, soak raw almonds in water, crush them, then filter out the solids. The resulting almond milk is creamy and somewhat sweet with a nutty flavour. It comes in both basic and flavoured varieties and is often low in fat, like soy milk.

Almond milk, particularly vanilla, has a pleasing flavour but produces less substance in ice cream compared to other non-dairy milks. It's a wonderful option for non-dairy ice cream bases when combined with thickeners to get a smooth and pleasing finish.

Coconut milk contains the greatest fat content of any non-dairy milk available. Coconut milk's high fat content produces creamy ice cream with a consistency similar to "regular" ice cream. Although coconut milk has a distinct flavour, it can be challenging to mask even with additional ingredients. Add Flavors to the ice cream base. If you don't enjoy coconut-flavoured foods, coconut milk may not be a suitable component.

Coconut milk is an excellent way to add a dash of coconut flavour to recipes. I love to use it in recipes to enhance the coconut flavour and make it more noticeable.

There are several coconut milk products available on the market. Both full-fat and low-fat coconut milk are typically packaged in cans. To prevent separation, shake them before use. For the creamiest ice cream, use full-fat coconut milk. However, low-fat milk can also be used. Coconut cream is a thicker variant of coconut milk made by filtering away the excess water. Coconut cream is more difficult to locate in supermarkets than coconut milk, but can be added to ice cream to create a richer, softer texture. Coconut cream is not to be confused with cream of coconut, which is a presweetened product used in tropical beverages like piña coladas and not for cooking.

Hemp milk and rice milk are **non-dairy alternatives** to soy milk that are prepared similarly. These milks are less commonly available than soy milks and, while popular, are not ideal for ice cream. Hemp milk Flavors can vary greatly between brands, with some having bitter overtones that may not be suitable for ice cream. Rice milk is less smooth than other non-dairy milks due to its watery consistency.

Sugar is a common ingredient in ice cream, sorbets, and granitas. It prevents ice crystals from forming, resulting in smoother ice cream and a sweeter foundation. Before freezing, some ice cream bases may appear overly sweet. However, freezing reduces the sweetness, resulting in a more balanced flavour. You can adjust the sugar content of a recipe based on your tastes.

If you start with extremely sweet fruit, you may be able to minimize the sugar in your sorbet. Please note that making large changes to the recipe may result in a somewhat different texture.

Agave syrup is a popular liquid sweetener derived from the agave plant. It is 1.5 times sweeter than cane sugar and can be easily included in ice cream bases due to its liquid consistency. Using agave syrup instead of sugar in a recipe may result in a different flavour due to its distinct flavour, which is not as neutral as sugar.

To substitute agave syrup for sugar in a recipe, begin by reducing the sweetness by 30%. Then, taste the base to see if it requires any additional sweetness, and add more agave as needed.

Maple syrup is a delicious sweetener with a distinct flavour. It is significantly sweeter than sugar and, like agave syrup, may be substituted in most recipes by using slightly less sugar. I don't advocate substituting maple syrup in any dish due to its strong flavour, which can dominate other ingredients.

Adding a tiny amount of **Alcohol** to ice cream helps avoid ice crystals and create a softer, more scoopable result. Add a tablespoon of neutral alcohol, such as vodka, to any of these recipes. Adding alcohol to ice cream does not significantly affect its texture; hence, it is best used to enhance flavour. To keep your ice cream alcohol-free, try adding a splash or omitting it from the recipes provided.

Non-dairy milks can be used to make dairy-free ice cream, but fruit-based frozen delights are more convenient and inherently dairy-free. Sorbets, prepared from fruit or juice and sugar, highlight the natural flavour of fruit in its brightest and most refreshing form. Sorbets are churned in ice cream makers, resulting in a scoopable consistency. Serve them as cones or sundaes with a fresh fruit topping.

Granitas, like sorbets, are made by combining fruit or juice with sugar. Granitas, which do not require an ice cream maker, are a popular option for individuals who prefer a low-tech approach to cooking.

Granitas To generate a gritty texture with huge ice crystals, freeze the mixture and then scrape it with a spoon or fork. Granitas often have a milder flavour than sorbets, but are still very refreshing.

Choosing an ice cream maker.

To make delicious homemade ice cream, whether dairy-free or not, consider investing in an ice cream maker. These machines can produce a batch of ice cream in the same amount of time as a pint of store-bought ice cream. Ice cream producers speedily chill and churn ice cream bases. Home ice cream producers quickly cool their bases and add air. Chilling quickly decreases ice crystals, resulting in smooth and creamy ice cream. Ice cream makers are available in several price ranges. With a number of sizes available, you can easily discover something that fits your kitchen and needs through comparison shopping.

There are three major types of ice cream producers. **A hand-churn ice cream maker** necessitates adding ice and salt to one chamber and a base to the other, then shaking or stirring as the base thickens. This is the most basic option.
This affordable machine produces softer ice cream, but it works well and provides a workout while churning each batch.

The most popular variety is the **canister ice cream maker.** To use this model, freeze the thick-walled canister ahead of time, and then pour the base into it to churn. Canister ice cream makers are small countertop appliances similar in size to food processors. You can use canister attachments with existing appliances, such stand mixers, to manufacture ice cream without purchasing a new machine. To use this sort of ice cream maker, plan ahead of time and freeze the canister at least 24 hours before usage. Otherwise, you may not be able to use it on short notice. Similar to hand-churn ice cream makers, this equipment can only produce one batch at a time.

The most expensive option is a **compressor ice cream maker**. The inbuilt compressor freezes your base as soon as you turn it on, eliminating the need for refreezing. Chilling the base before putting it to the machine is optional but can speed up the process.

This ice cream maker has the advantage of being ready to manufacture many batches quickly and without waiting time. This machine is not suitable for those who only make ice cream sometimes. However, if you frequently serve a large number of people, it can be useful.

Before using your ice cream maker, please sure to read the instructions carefully since each one may differ somewhat. Some ice cream makers shut off automatically once it reaches a certain thickness. When ice cream becomes thick and creamy, certain machines must be manually turned off.

Homemade ice cream is typically finished when it reaches a soft-serve consistency, as it does not freeze solid in an ice cream maker. To achieve a scoopable consistency, move the soft ice cream to a freezer-safe container and freeze for a few hours. Alternatively, you can consume the soft-serve version directly from the maker.

Before adding mix-ins, ice cream should be soft and freshly churned.

When churning your ice cream base, avoid adding nuts, chocolate chips, or fresh fruit since large chunks may cause the machine to become stuck.

After churning the ice cream, add caramel or fudge swirls made using store-bought sauces. If you add them during churning, they will be entirely folded into the ice cream, resulting in a new flavour rather than a swirl.

To avoid ice crystals, refrigerate ice cream in an airtight freezer container. Most ice creams can be scooped directly from the freezer, depending on its temperature. To soften ice cream, run the scoop under hot water before serving it.

To maintain the creamy consistency of ice cream, avoid melting the entire container too much, as this may cause it to refreeze with crystals. Store-bought ice creams typically have added emulsifiers and stabilizers to preserve texture for lengthy periods of storage, with the exception of excessive softening. Homemade ice cream is often consumed rapidly, so preserving it for more than a week is unlikely. Airtight containers can keep ice cream fresh for months in the freezer.

Ice cream can be made with or without an ice cream maker. Hand-stirring your ice cream is one option. To prepare, make your preferred ice cream base and pour into a large baking dish or basin. After 15-20 minutes of freezing, toss the mixture thoroughly with a fork.

This breaks any huge ice crystals that may be formed. Stir the ice cream every 15-20 minutes until it thickens and freezes. Add any desired mix-ins and serve immediately or store in an airtight container for later use. This method produces smoother ice cream than granita, but not as smooth as ice cream made using an ice cream maker.

Popsicles

Popsicles are a popular frozen dessert among children and adults.

Popsicles are both tasty and simple to create, requiring only a popsicle Mold. Popsicles can be made from any freezable liquid by pouring it into a Mold, and there are numerous Mold options available. A common popsicle mold may hold 2.5 ounces of liquid, but this is not an industry standard.

Therefore, your molds may create more or fewer popsicles. When filling popsicle molds with liquid, leave about a quarter inch at the top. Overfilling a mold with popsicles can cause them to overflow and create a sticky mess in the freezer as the bases expand during freezing.

If you don't have popsicle molds, you can make your own with a tiny cup or ice cube pan. Pour your liquid into a container and cover with plastic wrap or foil. To keep your popsicle sticks upright, poke them through the foil or plastic. Place the container in the freezer to set.

To unmold popsicles for serving, put them in warm water for a few seconds. To remove the popsicle from the mold, simply warm up the exterior. Avoid immersing your mold in water for too long, as it may cause the popsicle to melt.
Dip for a few seconds at a time, then check for a release. Repeat as needed.

Part 2:

The Recipes

The vegan ice cream recipes are categorized into three categories based on the milk used. The recipes for soy milk and almond milk ice cream are interchangeable due to their comparable production procedures. To achieve the finest results, use coconut milk instead of thickening agents.

Soy milk is the most often consumed non-dairy milk. Dried soybeans are mashed with water to produce a creamy liquid akin to low-fat milk. Vanilla soy milk, which is mildly sweetened and has a distinct vanilla flavour, is the ideal choice for these recipes. The extra vanilla enriches the other ingredients in the finished ice cream.

Vanilla Bean

Vanilla is the most popular ice cream flavour, including dairy-free options. This soy milk-based recipe is sure to become a hit at home. This recipe is simple and deliciously vanilla-flavoured. This dish can be enjoyed on its own or paired with any dessert.

3½ cups vanilla soy milk.

⅔ Cup Sugar

1 vanilla bean.

2 tablespoons cornstarch.

1. In a medium saucepan, combine 3 cups of soy milk and sugar. To extract the vanilla seeds, carefully slice the bean

in half lengthwise and scrape with a knife or spoon. Add to the milk and sugar mixture. Cook over medium heat, stirring occasionally, until the mixture reaches a simmer and the sugar dissolves.

2. Combine the remaining ½ cup soy milk and cornstarch in a small bowl. Add the cornstarch mixture to the simmering milk and sugar mixture and whisk until combined. Cook for 2-3 minutes, stirring regularly until the liquid thickens.

3. Transfer to a clean bowl, cover with plastic wrap, and let cool to room temperature. Refrigerate for at least 2-3 hours.

4. Follow manufacturer's instructions for making ice cream. Once churned, transfer the ice cream to a freezer-safe container and freeze for at least 2 hours before serving.

Makes approximately 1 pint.

Chocolates

Many people enjoy both vanilla and chocolate ice cream equally. This smooth ice cream has a surprisingly rich chocolate flavour, making it ideal for chocolate lovers.

3½ cups vanilla soy milk.

¾ cup sugar

1/2 cup cocoa powder.

1 tablespoon cornstarch

¼ teaspoon salt.

1 teaspoon of vanilla extract.

1. Mix 3 cups soy milk, sugar, and cocoa powder in a medium pot. Simmer over medium heat, whisking occasionally, until sugar and cocoa powder are dissolved.

2. Combine the remaining ½ cup milk and cornstarch in a small bowl. Add the cornstarch mixture to the simmering milk and sugar mixture, and whisk together.

Cook for 2-3 minutes, stirring regularly until the liquid thickens.

3. Remove from heat and mix in the salt and vanilla essence. Cool the mixture to room temperature in a clean basin, covered with plastic wrap. Refrigerate the mixture for at least 2-3 hours.

4. Follow the manufacturer's instructions to make the ice cream. After churning, transfer the ice cream to a freezer-safe container. Freeze for at least 2 hours before serving.

Makes approximately 1 pint.

Chocolate Chip

Chocolate chip ice cream is a flavour I never tire of! Making chocolate chips is key to a delicious chocolate chip ice cream recipe. Adding chopped chocolate to ice cream might make it difficult to chew. You won't taste much of the chocolate flavour because it doesn't melt in your mouth. Adding coconut oil to melted chocolate provides the ideal consistency for freezing.

3½ cups vanilla soy milk.

¾ cup sugar

2 tablespoons cornstarch.

2 teaspoons of vanilla extract.

3 ounces dark or semisweet chocolate, finely chopped.

2 teaspoons of coconut oil.

1. In a medium saucepan, combine 3 cups of soy milk and sugar. Cook over medium heat, whisking occasionally, until the mixture reaches a simmer and sugar dissolves.

2. Combine the remaining ½ cup milk and cornstarch in a small bowl. Add the cornstarch mixture to the simmering

milk and sugar mixture, and whisk together.

Cook for 2-3 minutes, stirring regularly until the liquid thickens.

3. Remove from heat and whisk in the vanilla essence. Transfer to a clean bowl, cover with plastic wrap, and let cool to room temperature. Refrigerate for at least 2–3 hours.

4. Follow the manufacturer's instructions to produce ice cream from the chilled mixture.

5. In a small microwave-safe bowl, combine the chocolate and coconut oil while the ice cream freezes. Microwave at medium speed for 30- to 40-second intervals, stirring regularly, until chocolate is melted and smooth.

6. After churning, drizzle the chocolate mixture into the ice cream and transfer to a freezer-safe container. Gently swirl to break up the chocolate ribbons. Combine all of the chocolate mixture.

Before serving, freeze for at least 2 hours to ensure firmness.

Makes approximately 1 pint.

Coffee

Soy milk is commonly used in coffee shops for lattes, so why not utilize it to make coffee ice cream? Instant espresso powder imparts a robust coffee flavour to the ice cream. If instant espresso powder is unavailable, substitute twice the amount with instant coffee powder, which is widely available in grocery shops.

3½ cups vanilla soy milk.

¾ cup sugar

2 tablespoons cornstarch.

2 teaspoons of vanilla extract.

Add 2½ teaspoons instant espresso or 5 tablespoons coffee powder.

1. In a medium saucepan, combine 3 cups of soy milk and sugar. Cook over medium heat, whisking occasionally, until the mixture reaches a simmer and sugar dissolves.

2. Combine the remaining ½ cup milk and cornstarch in a small bowl. Add the cornstarch mixture to the simmering milk and sugar mixture, and whisk together. Cook for 2-3 minutes, stirring regularly until the liquid thickens.

3. Remove from heat and mix in vanilla and instant espresso

powder. Transfer to a clean bowl, cover with plastic wrap, and cool to room temperature. Chill in the refrigerator for at least 2–3 hours.

4. Follow the manufacturer's instructions for making ice cream from the chilled mixture. Once churned, transfer the ice cream to a freezer-safe container and freeze for at least 2 hours before serving.

Makes approximately 1 pint.

Chocolate chip cookie dough.

When creating chocolate chip cookies, it's difficult to resist the urge to taste the raw dough straight from the bowl. This ice cream flavor features bits of chocolate chip cookie dough and extra chocolate chips, making it a must-try.

If you're a big fan of cookie dough, make a double batch and sprinkle it on top while serving.

3½ cups vanilla soy milk.

¾ cup sugar

2 tablespoons cornstarch.

2 teaspoons of vanilla extract.

Make 1 batch of vegan chocolate chip cookie dough chunks (recipe below).

1/2 cup small chocolate chips.

1. In a medium saucepan, combine 3 cups soy milk and sugar. Cook over medium heat, whisking occasionally, until the mixture reaches a simmer and sugar dissolves.

2. Combine the remaining ½ cup milk and cornstarch in a small bowl. Add the cornstarch mixture to the simmering milk and sugar mixture, and whisk together. Cook for 2-3 minutes, stirring regularly, until the liquid thickens.

3. Remove from heat and whisk in the vanilla essence. Transfer to a clean bowl, cover with plastic wrap, and let cool to room temperature. Refrigerate for at least 2–3 hours.

4. Follow the manufacturer's instructions to produce ice cream from the chilled mixture. After churning the ice cream, add Vegan Chocolate Chip Cookie Dough Chunks and chocolate chips. Transfer the ice cream to a freezer-safe container and freeze for at least 2 hours before serving.

Makes approximately 1 quart of

Vegan chocolate chip cookie dough chunks.

⅓ cup vegan margarine or shortening at room temperature.

1/2 cup brown sugar, packed.

½ teaspoon vanilla extract.

¼ teaspoon salt

1 tablespoon of soy milk.

1/2 cup all-purpose flour.

1/2 cup small chocolate chips.

1. Cream together the margarine and brown sugar until smooth.

Combine the vanilla extract, salt, and soy milk. Mix in the flour until the dough comes together. Stir in the chocolate chips.

2. Form the dough into small, almond-sized balls. Refrigerate until ready for use.

Makes approximately 1 cup.

Strawberry

Strawberry ice cream, despite its simplicity, is one of the most beloved tastes of all time. Fresh strawberry ice cream is a summertime must-have dessert. Pair with a slice of cake and fresh berries for a refreshing strawberry shortcake.

3 cups of fresh strawberries.

1½ cups vanilla soy milk.

½ cup sugar

¼ teaspoon almond extract.

1/2 cup finely chopped strawberries.

1. Mix strawberries, soy milk, sugar, and almond extract in a food processor or blender. Blend until smooth and sugar is completely dissolved.

2. Place in a big bowl and cover with plastic wrap. Refrigerate for approximately 2 hours, or until cool.

3. Follow the manufacturer's instructions for making ice cream from the chilled mixture. After churning, transfer the ice cream to a freezer-safe container and fold in finely

chopped strawberries. Freeze for at least two hours before serving.

Makes approximately 1 pint.

Maple Syrup

When I first tried maple syrup ice cream, I was surprised because I had not previously linked it with frozen treats. The syrup had a toffee-like flavour and tasted even better cold than when served with pancakes. For optimal results, choose dark amber or Grade B maple syrup, as they have a stronger maple flavour than lighter grades.

3½ cups vanilla soy milk.

1/2 cup grade B or dark amber maple syrup

2 tablespoons cornstarch.

1 teaspoon of vanilla extract.

1. In a medium saucepan, combine 3 cups of soy milk and maple syrup. Cook over medium heat, stirring occasionally, until the mixture reaches a simmer and maple syrup dissolves.

2. Combine the remaining ½ cup milk and cornstarch in a small bowl. Whisk the cornstarch mixture into the

simmering milk and maple syrup until well combined. Cook for 2-3 minutes, stirring regularly until the liquid thickens. Whisk in the vanilla extract.

3. Remove from heat, transfer to a clean bowl, wrap in plastic, and cool to room temperature. Refrigerate for at least 2-3 hours.

4. Follow the manufacturer's instructions for making ice cream from the chilled mixture. Once churned, transfer the ice cream to a freezer-safe container and freeze for at least 2 hours before serving.

Makes approximately 1 pint.

Chai tea

Inspired by the chai tea latte, this ice cream flavour is both sweet and spicy. It is recommended to begin with a high-quality chai tea concentrate.

These are carefully designed to offer maximum spiciness and are already sweetened. This chai tea latté is lightly sweetened with agave syrup.

1½ cup chai tea concentrate

1½ cups vanilla soy milk.

¼ cup agave syrup

1 teaspoon of vanilla extract.

1. In a large bowl, add chai tea, soy milk, agave, and vanilla. Whisk well. To taste, add more agave syrup.

2. Cover bowl with plastic wrap and refrigerate for 1 hour.

3. Follow the manufacturer's instructions for making ice cream from the chilled mixture. Once churned, transfer the ice cream to a freezer-safe container and freeze for at least 2 hours before serving.

Makes approximately 1 pint.

Non-dairy drinkers often prefer almond milk to soy milk. It has a mellow, nutty flavour that is more subtle than soy milk. Almond milk, like soy milk, is available in both unsweetened and sweetened varieties. Lightly sweetened vanilla almond milk adds flavour to these recipes and is an excellent pantry staple for quick ice cream creation.

Cherry Chocolate Chip

This flavour resembles a popular cherry-studded ice cream from a well-known brand. Almond milk's mild flavour pairs well with cherries. This dish works best with frozen or jarred cherries. They are available year-round and slightly more tender than fresh cherries, making them simpler to incorporate into ice cream and providing more juice to flavour the base.

3½ cups of vanilla almond milk.

¾ cup sugar

2 tablespoons cornstarch.

1 teaspoon of vanilla extract.

1 teaspoon almond extract.

3 ounces dark or semisweet chocolate, finely chopped.

2 teaspoons of coconut oil.

1½ cups canned or frozen dark cherries, defrosted (continued on the following page).

1. Mix 3 cups almond milk and sugar in a medium saucepan. Cook over medium heat, whisking occasionally, until mixture reaches a simmer and sugar dissolves.

2. Combine the remaining ½ cup milk and cornstarch in a small bowl. Add the cornstarch mixture to the simmering milk and sugar mixture, and whisk together. Cook for 2-3 minutes, stirring regularly until the liquid thickens.

3. Remove from heat and mix in the vanilla and almond extracts.

Transfer to a clean bowl, wrap with plastic wrap, and cool to room temperature. Refrigerate for at least 2-3 hours.

4. Follow the manufacturer's instructions to produce ice cream from the chilled mixture.

5. In a small microwave-safe bowl, combine the chocolate and coconut oil while the ice cream freezes. Microwave at medium speed for 30- to 40-second intervals, stirring

regularly, until chocolate is melted and smooth.

6. After churning the ice cream, fold in the cherries and drizzle with the chocolate mixture. Transfer to a freezer-safe container and gently swirl to create ribbons of chocolate that will break up. Freeze for at least 2 hours before serving. Makes approximately 1 pint.

Peanut butter and bananas

The combination of salty peanut butter and sweet bananas works well in a sandwich, so it makes sense to use it in ice cream too. This recipe is simple and delicious, especially with the creamy peanut butter.

Three large, ripe bananas

1 cup of vanilla almond milk.

1 cup of creamy peanut butter.

1/2 cup agave syrup.

Ingredients: 2 tablespoons vanilla extract, ¼ teaspoon salt.

1. Blend together bananas, almond milk, peanut butter, agave, vanilla, and salt until creamy. Transfer to a bowl, cover with plastic wrap, and chill for 2 hours.

2. Follow the manufacturer's instructions to produce ice cream from the chilled mixture. Once churned, transfer the ice cream to a freezer-safe container. Freeze until hard, at least 2 hours before serving.

Makes approximately 1 pint.

Mocha Almond Fudge

This ice cream, a Favorite of my father's, combines coffee, chocolate, and almonds. When he originally told me about this combo, which he enjoyed at a popular ice cream chain, I wondered if there were too many tastes involved. The Flavors complement each other well, leaving you wanting more.

3½ cups of vanilla almond milk.

¾ cup sugar and 2 teaspoons instant espresso powder.

2 tablespoons cornstarch.

2 teaspoons of vanilla extract.

3 ounces of roughly chopped dark or semisweet chocolate.

1/2 cup toasted slivered almonds.

¾ cup Dark Chocolate Fudge Sauce

1. Mix 3 cups almond milk, sugar, and espresso powder in a medium pot. Cook over medium heat, stirring occasionally, until mixture reaches a simmer and sugar dissolves.

2. Combine the remaining ½ cup milk and cornstarch in a small bowl. When the milk/sugar mixture reaches a simmer, add the cornstarch mixture and whisk until combined. Cook for 2-3 minutes, stirring regularly until the liquid thickens.

3. Remove from heat and stir in vanilla essence and chocolate until fully dissolved. Transfer to a clean bowl, cover with plastic wrap, and let cool to room temperature. Refrigerate for at least 2 to 3 hours.

4. Follow the manufacturer's instructions to produce ice cream from the chilled mixture. After churning the ice cream, add toasted almonds and drizzle with chocolate fudge sauce before transferring to a freezer-safe container, producing ribbons of chocolate. Freeze for at least 2 hours before serving.

This makes approximately 1 pint.

Banana with Toasted Pecan

Toasted nuts enhance the flavour of banana bread and ice cream. This breakfast pastry-inspired ice cream pairs well with pecans, which have a natural sweetness that complements the almond milk used in the recipe.

Untoasted 1½ cup coarsely chopped pecans

2 huge ripe medium bananas

1½ cups vanilla almond milk

⅔ cup sugar and 1 teaspoon vanilla essence.

1/2 teaspoon ground cinnamon

1. Place pecans in a large skillet and fry over medium-low heat.

Cook pecans till golden brown, stirring carefully and regularly. Remove the heat.

2. In a blender or food processor, combine bananas, almond milk, sugar, vanilla, cinnamon, and ½ cup toasted nuts. Process until smooth and sugar is dissolved. To remove toasted pecans, pour through a fine sieve into a big basin.

3. Cover with plastic wrap and chill for 2 hours.

4. Follow the manufacturer's instructions to produce ice cream from the chilled mixture.

5. While ice cream is churning, coarsely chop the remaining

pecans.

6. After churning, transfer the ice cream to a freezer-safe container and fold in the remaining roasted pecans.

Before serving, freeze for at least 2 hours to ensure firmness.

Makes approximately 1 pint.

Horchata

Horchata, a sweet and spicy drink, is popular in Spanish-speaking and Latin American countries. It can be created with a variety of nuts and grains. Mexican horchata, traditionally made with almonds and rice, can be transformed into a delectable dessert with some imagination.

6 cups of vanilla almond milk.

1 cup of basmati rice (or other short-grain rice).

Ingredients: ¾ cup sugar, 1/2 teaspoon ground cinnamon.

1 teaspoon of vanilla extract.

1. Pour almond milk into a large mixing dish. Grind basmati rice in a spice or coffee grinder to a fine, sand-like consistency. Combine rice, sugar, cinnamon, and vanilla in almond milk. Cover and leave at room temperature for 10–12 hours.

2. Strain the pounded rice from the milk mixture into a large basin or pitcher using cheesecloth. Refrigerate for at least one hour, or until thoroughly cooled.

3. Follow the manufacturer's instructions to produce ice cream from the chilled mixture. Once churned, transfer the ice cream to a freezer-safe container. Freeze until hard, at least 2 hours before serving.

Makes approximately 1 pint.

Coconut milk has a naturally sweet and fuller texture than other non-dairy milks, making it ideal for use in recipes. Cooking fresh coconut with water releases its natural fat and taste. Full-fat coconut milk is ideal for rich ice cream, while low-fat coconut milk is suitable for lighter desserts.

Vanilla and toasted coconut

If you've never tried vanilla and coconut combined, this ice cream recipe is a must-try. This recipe boasts a delicious vanilla taste and includes toasted coconut for texture and flavour. Use either sweetened or unsweetened shredded coconut for best results, depending on availability.

1 cup shredded coconut, sweet or unsweetened

3½ cup unsweetened coconut milk

¾ cup sugar

1 tablespoon of vanilla extract.

1. Finely chop the shredded coconut and lay it in a big skillet. Cook on low heat until the coconut toasts and turns a light golden color. Cook the coconut until equally golden brown,

stirring gently and constantly. Set it aside to cool.

2. Mix together coconut milk, sugar, and vanilla in a food processor or blender. Blend until smooth and sugar is completely dissolved.

3. Place in a big basin and cover with plastic wrap. Refrigerate for approximately one hour, or until cool.

4. Follow manufacturer's instructions for making ice cream. After churning, transfer the ice cream to a freezer-safe container and add toasted coconut. Before serving, freeze for at least 2 hours to ensure firmness.

Makes approximately 1 quart

Cookies 'n' Cream

Making a vegan version of cookies 'n' cream ice cream is simple, given Oreos and similar brands are already vegan. For this recipe, I recommend using a combination of coconut and soy milk. The coconut adds richness to the ice cream, while the soy milk balances it out with a subtle vanilla flavour.

1½ cup unsweetened coconut milk

2 cups of vanilla soy milk.

⅔ Cup Sugar

2 teaspoons of vanilla extract.

1½ cups crushed Oreo cookies.

1. Mix together coconut milk, soy milk, sugar, and vanilla in a food processor or blender. Blend until smooth and sugar is completely dissolved.

2. Place in a big bowl and cover with plastic wrap. Refrigerate for approximately one hour, or until cool.

3. Follow manufacturer's instructions for making ice cream. After churning, transfer the ice cream to a freezer-safe container and add crumbled Oreo cookies. Before serving, freeze for at least 2 hours to ensure firmness.

Makes approximately 1 pint.

Coconut Mint Chocolate Chip

Mint chocolate chip ice cream is pleasant but not particularly intriguing. Adding shredded coconut to ice cream made with coconut milk gives a unique flavour to this variation of mint chocolate chip ice cream, while it is not required. For some, mint chocolate chip ice cream is not complete without a little green hue. If you prefer it this way, add a few drops of green food colouring.

3½ cups unsweetened coconut milk

¾ cup sugar

2 teaspoons of vanilla extract.

1½ tablespoons peppermint extract ¼ teaspoon green food colouring (optional)

3 ounces dark or semisweet chocolate, finely chopped

2 teaspoons of coconut oil.

1/2 cup shredded coconut (sweetened or unsweetened)

1. In a food processor or blender, combine coconut milk, sugar, vanilla, peppermint, and green food colouring (optional). Blend until smooth and sugar is completely dissolved.

Coconut milk ice creams (43)

2. Place in a big bowl and cover with plastic wrap.

Refrigerate for approximately one hour, or until cool.

3. Follow the manufacturer's instructions for making ice cream.

4. In a small microwave-safe bowl, combine the chocolate

and coconut oil while the ice cream freezes. Microwave at medium speed for 30- to 40-second intervals, stirring regularly, until chocolate is melted and smooth.

5. After churning, drop the chocolate mixture into the ice cream and transfer to a freezer-safe container. Stir gently to break up the chocolate ribbons. Stir in the shredded coconut after thoroughly incorporating the chocolate mixture. Freeze for at least two hours before serving.

Makes approximately 1 pint.

Coconut Chocolate

Chocolate and coconut make an excellent mix, as evidenced by a walk down the candy aisle. The coconut's natural sweetness complements dark chocolate and adds creaminess. This ice cream recipe combines cocoa powder with instant coffee powder to create a rich chocolate flavour with a hint of coconut.

3½ cups unsweetened coconut milk

¾ cup sugar

1/2 cup cocoa powder.

1 teaspoon of instant coffee powder.

1 teaspoon of vanilla extract.

1. Mix coconut milk, sugar, cocoa powder, coffee powder, and vanilla in a food processor or blender. Blend until smooth and sugar is completely dissolved.

2. Place in a big bowl and cover with plastic wrap. Refrigerate for approximately one hour, or until cool.

3. Follow the manufacturer's instructions for making ice cream. After churning, transfer the ice cream to a freezer-safe container and add toasted coconut. Before serving, freeze for at least 2 hours to ensure firmness.

Makes approximately 1 pint.

Coconut Pumpkin Spice

One year, around Thanksgiving, I was handed a slice of coconut pumpkin pie and recognized what a terrific flavour combination. The ice cream has a tinge of coconut flavour from coconut milk but is mostly flavoured with pumpkin and pumpkin pie spices.

This recipe is a delicious alternative to classic pies for fall and winter desserts.

3 cups unsweetened coconut milk.

1 cup pumpkin puree.

⅓ cup maple syrup.

2 tablespoons brown sugar.

3 tablespoons molasses.

1/2 teaspoon ground cinnamon

1 teaspoon ground ginger.

1/4 teaspoon ground cloves.

1/4 teaspoon salt.

1 teaspoon of vanilla extract.

1. Mix coconut milk, pumpkin, maple syrup, sugar, molasses, cinnamon, ginger, cloves, salt, and vanilla in a food processor or blender. Blend until smooth and sugar is completely dissolved.

2. Place in a big bowl and cover with plastic wrap. Refrigerate for approximately one hour, or until cool.

3. Follow the manufacturer's instructions for making ice cream. Once churned, transfer the ice cream to a freezer-safe container. Freeze for a minimum of 2 hours before serving.

This makes approximately 1 quart

Coconut mango rice.

This flavour was inspired by my Favorite Thai delicacy, sticky rice with mango. The base consists of delectable coconut rice pudding. Rice pudding can transform into delicious ice cream due to its soft texture and flavour. After churning, fold in the diced mango to ensure even distribution throughout each bite.

1/2 cup uncooked short-grain rice.

¾ cup sugar

2½ cups water

2 cups of unsweetened coconut milk.

2 teaspoons of vanilla extract.

One large, ripe mango, peeled and finely chopped

1. In a medium saucepan, combine rice, sugar, and water. Begin by bringing the mixture to a boil and stirring to dissolve the sugar. Then, reduce to a simmer and cook for about 45 minutes, or until the liquid is completely absorbed.
2. Add coconut milk and cook rice over low heat. Cook for 20-30 minutes until rice is extremely soft. Stir in the vanilla.

Transfer pudding to a large bowl, cover, and chill for at least 4 hours or until cold.

3. Follow the manufacturer's instructions for making ice cream. After churning, transfer the ice cream to a freezer-safe container and fold in diced mango. Before serving, freeze for at least 2 hours to ensure firmness.

Makes approximately 1 pint.

Coconut, raspberries, and lime

This ice cream's light pink tint adds to its allure, making it difficult to guess the flavour until you take a bite. This dessert is sweet with a tinge of acidity, combining three tastes that complement each other perfectly. Adding fresh lime juice to coconut milk does not curdle it, allowing for a smoother ice cream foundation when blended.

3 cups unsweetened coconut milk.

¾ cup sugar

2 cups of fresh raspberries.

1/2 cup freshly squeezed lime juice.

1 tablespoon of lime zest.

1/2 cup toasted coconut.

1. Mix together coconut milk, sugar, raspberries, lime juice, and zest in a food processor or blender. Blend until smooth and sugar is completely dissolved.

2. Strain the mixture into a large basin to remove the raspberry seeds. Cover with plastic wrap. Refrigerate for approximately 1 hour.

3. Follow the manufacturer's instructions for making ice cream. After churning, transfer the ice cream to a freezer-safe container and add toasted coconut. Before serving, freeze for at least 2 hours to ensure firmness.

Makes approximately 1 pint.

SORBETS AND GRANITAS are refreshing fruit-based desserts ideal for hot days. These treats satisfy your sweet taste, similar to ice cream, but offer a refreshing alternative. To enhance the flavour of your sorbets and granitas, use fresh, in-season fruits. Alternatively, frozen fruits can be used year-round.

Bittersweet Chocolate Sorbet.

This dark chocolate sorbet provides a luscious chocolate dessert without the need for dairy or other ingredients. This is a highly addicting way to satisfy your chocolate cravings. To maximize flavour, use high-quality dark chocolate for this recipe.

3½ cups of water.

1½ cup sugar

1 cup unsweetened cocoa powder.

1 teaspoon of instant coffee powder.

2 oz. dark chocolate, finely chopped

2 tablespoons vanilla extract,

¼ teaspoon salt.

1. Mix water, sugar, cocoa powder, and instant coffee in a medium pot. Cook over medium heat, whisking occasionally, until the sugar and cocoa powder dissolve completely.

2. Remove from heat and mix in the dark chocolate, vanilla, and salt.

Stir carefully until the dark chocolate has melted completely.

3. Transfer to a clean bowl, cover with plastic wrap, and cool until room temperature. Refrigerate for at least 2–3 hours.

4. Follow the manufacturer's instructions for making ice cream from the chilled mixture. Once churned, transfer the ice cream to a freezer-safe container and freeze for at least 2 hours before serving.

Makes approximately 1 pint.

Blueberry Sorbet

Blueberries are sometimes overlooked in frozen sweets compared to strawberries and raspberries. However, their jammy texture makes for a sweet and delightful sorbet. This recipe uses fresh blueberries and turns a beautiful magenta hue after churning.

4 cups of fresh or frozen blueberries, defrosted

Combine ¾ cup sugar with 1 cup water.

2 teaspoons of vanilla extract.

2 teaspoons of Cointreau or other orange liqueur.

1. Mix blueberries, sugar, water, vanilla, and Cointreau in a food processor or blender. Blend until smooth and sugar is completely dissolved.

2. Place in a big bowl and cover with plastic wrap. Refrigerate for approximately one hour, or until cool.

3. Follow the manufacturer's instructions for making ice cream from the chilled mixture. Once churned, transfer the ice cream to a freezer-safe container. Freeze until hard, at least 2 hours before serving.

Makes approximately 1 pint.

Peach Melba Sorbet

A peach melba is a classic dish made with peaches, raspberries, and vanilla ice cream, similar to an ice cream sundae. This luscious sorbet, inspired by melba, features sweet peaches and tangy raspberries. To enhance the peach flavor, I use vanilla extract to mimic the taste of vanilla ice cream and peach schnapps.

5-6 big, juicy peaches.

1 cup water. 1 cup sugar.

2 teaspoons of vanilla extract.

2 tablespoons peach schnapps (optional) 2 cups of fresh raspberries.

1. Peel and pit the peaches. Cut peaches into medium bits, yielding approximately 3½ cups.

2. In a large pot, combine water and sugar. Cook over medium heat and whisk until sugar melts. Simmer peaches, stirring periodically, until soft.

Remove the heat. If using, stir in the vanilla and peach schnapps.

3. Place in a big basin and cover with plastic wrap.

Refrigerate until cool, about 2 to 3 hours.

4. Follow the manufacturer's instructions for making ice

cream from the chilled mixture. After churning the sorbet, fold in fresh raspberries until evenly distributed. Transfer to a freezer-safe container and freeze for at least 2 hours before serving.

Makes approximately 1 pint.

Tangerine & Olive Oil Sorbet

This sorbet is a go-to recipe when I have an abundance of tangerines to juice. Oranges pair well with olive oil in both savory and sweet meals. The oil unexpectedly provides a refined accent to the spicy tangerine base. To balance the tartness of the juice, this sorbet recipe recommends adding a small amount of added sugar.

3½ cups of freshly squeezed tangerine juice.

⅓ cup fresh squeezed lemon juice

1½ cup sugar

3 tablespoons of good-quality olive oil.

1. Mix tangerine juice, lemon juice, and sugar in a medium saucepan. Bring to a simmer and whisk constantly to dissolve the sugar. Remove from heat and whisk in olive oil.

2. Place in a big bowl and cover with plastic wrap.

Refrigerate until cool, about 2 to 3 hours.

3. Prepare the cooled mixture in an ice cream maker according to the manufacturer's instructions. After churning, transfer the sorbet to a freezer-safe container. Freeze for at least 2 hours before serving.

This makes approximately 1 pint

Strawberry Watermelon Sorbet

Strawberry and watermelon are the quintessential summer Flavors. Combine these two juicy fruits for a wonderful summer treat that's even better when frozen. To brighten the tastes of the sorbet, I always add a splash of lemon juice. For an adult treat, pair this with champagne.

6 cups of watermelon, chopped into large bits

2 cups of chopped strawberries

⅔ Cup Sugar, 2 teaspoons of lemon juice.

1. Mix watermelon, strawberries, sugar, and lemon juice in a food processor or blender. Blend until smooth and sugar is completely dissolved.

2. Place in a big bowl and cover with plastic wrap. Refrigerate for approximately one hour, or until cool.

3. Follow the manufacturer's instructions for making ice cream from the chilled mixture. Once churned, transfer the sorbet to a freezer-safe container and freeze for at least 2 hours before serving.

Makes approximately 1 pint.

Spiced Cranberry Sorbet

Cranberry juice is a delicious drink that I enjoy all year, but due to its frequent use in holiday recipes, I associate it more with the holidays.

This spiced cranberry sorbet tastes like mulled wine and is packed with spices. To enhance the flavour of the sorbet, I add orange zest, Cointreau, or another orange liqueur.

4 cups cranberry juice.

1 tablespoon of orange zest.

1 tablespoon of lemon zest.

Six cinnamon sticks.

Twelve whole cloves.

1 teaspoon ground allspice.

1 cup sugar.

Optional: ¼ cup Cointreau or other orange liqueur.

1. Mix cranberry juice, orange and lemon zests, cinnamon sticks, cloves, allspice, and sugar in a big pot. Cook over medium heat, stirring until sugar dissolves.

Bring to a boil. Remove from heat, cover, and steep for at least an hour.

2. Strain the liquid to remove the zest, spices, and cinnamon sticks. Stir in Cointreau, if desired.

3. Place in a big basin and cover with plastic wrap. Refrigerate until cool, about 2 to 3 hours.

4. Follow the manufacturer's instructions for making ice cream from the chilled mixture. Once churned, transfer the sorbet to a freezer-safe container and freeze for at least 2 hours before serving.

Makes approximately 1 pint.

Meyer Lemon Granita.

Meyer lemons are a hybrid fruit that has the flavor of lemons but lacks the acidity. Meyer lemons are ideal for making sorbets and granitas because they require less sugar than regular lemon juice. To make this recipe without Meyer lemons, use equal parts lemon juice and water, with a slight increase in sugar.

1 cup water.

¾ cup sugar

3 cups Meyer lemon juice, freshly squeezed.

1 tablespoon of Meyer lemon zest.

1. In a small saucepan, combine water and sugar. Bring to a simmer and stir until sugar is dissolved.
Remove from heat and combine sugar syrup, Meyer lemon juice, and zest.
2. Transfer to a flat, shallow dish, like a 9-by-9-inch baking or casserole dish, and freeze.
3. Stir granita every 20–25 minutes to evenly disperse the ice crystals. After granita has frozen for 3-4 hours or overnight, use a large spoon to scrape into serving dishes.
Makes approximately 1 pint.

Coffee granita

On a hot day, a bowl of coffee granita is more refreshing than iced coffee. This version has a strong coffee flavour with a perfect balance of sweetness. To make a simple variation, add a half teaspoon of cinnamon to the sugar syrup instead of only using coffee.

1 cup water.

1 cup sugar.

3 cups of strong coffee.

1. In a small saucepan, combine water and sugar. Bring to a simmer and stir until sugar is dissolved.

Remove from heat and stir in the coffee.

2. Transfer to a flat, shallow dish, like a 9-by-9-inch baking or casserole dish, and freeze.

3. Stir granita every 20–25 minutes to evenly disperse the ice crystals. After granita has frozen for 3-4 hours or overnight, use a large spoon to scrape into serving dishes.

Makes approximately 1 pint.

Blood orange granita.

Blood oranges are recognized for their deep crimson hue and unique taste. Making granita with them creates a visually appealing and delicious dessert. To achieve optimal results, use freshly squeezed juice in this recipe. The granita has a noticeable flavour change.

1 cup water.

¾ cup sugar

3 cups blood orange juice, freshly squeezed.

1 tablespoon of blood orange zest.

1. In a small saucepan, combine water and sugar. Bring to a simmer and stir until sugar is dissolved.
Remove from heat and mix sugar syrup, blood orange juice, and zest.

2. Transfer to a flat, shallow dish, like a 9-by-9-inch baking or casserole dish, and freeze.

3. Stir granita every 20–25 minutes to evenly disperse the ice crystals. After granita has frozen for 3-4 hours or overnight, use a large spoon to scrape into serving dishes.

Makes approximately 1 pint.

Pineapple granita reminds me of Hawaii's shave ice.

This shave ice (not shaved ice) is produced with finely ground ice and exotic tropical syrups. This pineapple granita is simple to make at home and has a sweet tropical flavour.

4 cups roughly chopped pineapple

1 cup water.

¾ cup sugar

1. Mix pineapple, water, and sugar in a food processor or blender. Blend until smooth and sugar is completely dissolved.

2. Transfer to a flat, shallow dish, like a 9-by-9-inch baking or casserole dish, and freeze.

3. Stir granita every 20–25 minutes to evenly disperse the ice crystals. After granita has frozen for 3-4 hours or overnight, use a large spoon to scrape it onto serving dishes.

Makes approximately 1 pint.

Tart Cherry Granita

Cherry popsicles were a childhood Favorite, but as I grew older, I realized they didn't taste like genuine cherries. This granita is created with actual cherry juice, which gives it its vivid red colour. While it won't turn your mouth and tongue red like childhood popsicles, it will delight your taste buds with a hint of authentic cherry flavour.

4 cups of tart cherry juice.

1 cup sugar.

1. In a small saucepan, combine 2 cups of cherry juice and sugar. Bring to a simmer and stir until sugar is dissolved. Remove from heat and mix in the remaining 2 cups of cherry juice.

2. Transfer to a flat, shallow dish, like a 9-by-9-inch baking or casserole dish, and freeze.

3. Stir granita every 20–25 minutes to evenly disperse the ice crystals. After granita has frozen for 3-4 hours or overnight, use a large spoon to scrape into serving dishes.

This makes approximately 1 quart

Honeydew & Mint Granita

Honeydew melons are a perfect base for granitas due to their high-water content and delicate natural sweetness. This granita combines the honeyed flavour of honeydew with a hint of mint, creating a refreshing yet sweet treat.

8 cups honeydew, sliced into big bits.

½ cup sugar

2 tablespoons of lime juice.

10–12 mint leaves

1. Mix honeydew, sugar, lime juice, and mint in a food processor or blender. Blend until smooth and sugar is completely dissolved.

2. Transfer to a flat, shallow dish, like a 9-by-9-inch baking or casserole dish, and freeze.

3. Stir granita every 20–25 minutes to evenly disperse the ice crystals. After granita has frozen for 3-4 hours or overnight, use a large spoon to scrape into serving dishes.

Makes approximately 1 pint.

Pears and cinnamon Granita

Granita is a popular summer dessert that is both light and refreshing. They're a light and refreshing way to end a heavy meal, making them ideal for the holidays, especially in cold weather. This granita, created with pear juice and a dash of cinnamon, embodies the Christmas spirit in a unique package.

4 cups pear juice.

1 teaspoon ground cinnamon.

¼ teaspoon allspice.

1 teaspoon of vanilla extract.

1 cup sugar.

1. In a small saucepan, combine 2 cups pear juice with cinnamon, allspice, vanilla, and sugar. Bring to a simmer and stir until sugar is fully dissolved. Remove from heat and add the remaining 2 cups pear juice.

2. Transfer to a flat, shallow dish, like a 9-by-9-inch baking or casserole dish, and freeze.

3. Stir granita every 20–25 minutes to evenly disperse the ice crystals. After granita has frozen for 3-4 hours or overnight, use a large spoon to scrape into serving dishes.

Makes approximately 1 pint.

People of all ages enjoy popsicles. These frozen delights are ideal for a quick afternoon snack after school or work. Make a batch ahead of time to satisfy cravings whenever they arise.

Dark Chocolate Pudding Pops.

Two out of every three children chose chocolate pudding pops over vanilla. These pops, made with cocoa powder and dark chocolate, are sure to satisfy any chocolate fan.

2½ cups vanilla soy milk.

⅔ Cup Sugar

3 tablespoons chocolate powder.

3 tablespoons cornstarch.

1 teaspoon salt.

1 teaspoon of vanilla extract.

1 ½ ounces finely chopped dark chocolate.

1. Mix 2 cups soy milk, sugar, and cocoa powder in a medium pot. Cook over medium heat, stirring occasionally, until the mixture reaches a simmer and the sugar dissolves.

73 | *Vegan Frozen Desserts Mastery: 50 Plant-Based Ice Creams, Sorbets & Granitas*

2. Combine the remaining ½ cup soy milk, cornstarch, and salt in a small basin. Add the cornstarch mixture to the simmering milk and sugar mixture, and whisk together.

Cook for 2-3 minutes, stirring regularly, until the pudding thickens.

3. Remove from heat, and whisk in the vanilla and chopped chocolate.

Stir until the chocolate has melted into the pudding.

4. Transfer to a clean bowl, cover with plastic wrap, and cool until room temperature. Pour the chilled mixture into popsicle molds and freeze for at least 6 hours or overnight to solidify.

Makes 6–8 popsicles.

Vanilla pudding pops

This popsicle recipe recalls a childhood Favorite: pudding pops. The recipe uses vegan vanilla pudding, similar to ice cream, but with added cornstarch to achieve the desired consistency. This dish is delicious, both fresh from the pan and frozen.

2½ cups vanilla soy milk.

½ cup sugar

5 tablespoons cornstarch.

1 teaspoon salt.

1 teaspoon of vanilla extract.

1. In a medium saucepan, combine 2 cups of soy milk and sugar. Cook over medium heat, stirring occasionally, until mixture reaches a simmer and sugar dissolves.

2. Combine the remaining ½ cup milk, cornstarch, and salt in a small bowl. Add the cornstarch mixture to the simmering milk and sugar mixture, and whisk together. Cook for 2-3 minutes, stirring regularly, until the pudding thickens.

3. Remove from heat and mix in vanilla. Transfer to a clean bowl, cover with plastic wrap, and let cool to room temperature. Chill the mixture before freezing it in popsicle molds for at least 6 hours or overnight until solid.

Makes 6–8 popsicles.

Banana Pudding Pops.

Inspired by banana cream pie, these pops have a luscious banana and vanilla flavour. The popsicles feature a sprinkling of Graham cracker crumbs at the base, reminiscent of the pie's crust.

Two ripe medium bananas.

3/4 cup vanilla soy milk

⅓ Cup Sugar

1 teaspoon vanilla extract.

2-3 teaspoons of Graham cracker crumbs.

1. Blend or process bananas, soy milk, sugar, and vanilla until smooth and sugar is dissolved.

2. Fill popsicle molds and top with Graham cracker crumbs, about a teaspoon each. Freeze for at least 6 hours (or overnight) until solid.

Makes 6–8 popsicles.

Cherry Lemonade Pops

These two-layer pops must be frozen in two processes. First, freeze the lemon layer at the bottom of the popsicle. Then, insert the stick and add the cherry layer. To get the best results, be near your freezer when making them. The end result is well worth it!

1 cup of cherry juice.

⅔ Cup Sugar

1/2 cup lemon juice.

½ cup water

1. Mix cherry juice and ¼ cup sugar in a small pot.
Cook on low heat, stirring occasionally, until sugar is fully dissolved. Set it aside to cool.

2. In another small pot, mix lemon juice, water, and remaining sugar. Cook on low heat, stirring occasionally, until sugar is fully dissolved. Set it aside to cool.

3. Fill popsicle molds halfway with lemon mixture and freeze for 3-4 hours. Fill the molds with the remaining cherry mixture, then insert sticks and lids.

Freeze for at least 6 hours, preferably overnight, to solidify.

Makes 6–8 popsicles.

Blueberry Balsamic Pops.

Balsamic vinegar is sometimes overlooked as a dessert ingredient, but it may enhance many berry recipes. The overwhelming sweetness complements the naturally sweet berries, while the powerful acidity highlights the sweetness. Simply put, it enhances the flavor of the blueberries and elevates the pops to a level above what you'd expect from an ice cream truck.

12 ounces of fresh blueberries.

⅓ Cup Sugar

2 tablespoons of water.

2 teaspoons of balsamic vinegar.

1. In a blender or food processor, combine blueberries, sugar, water, and vinegar. Process until smooth and sugar dissolved.

2. Pour into popsicle molds and freeze for 6 hours or overnight until solid.

Makes 6–8 popsicles.

Mojito Pops

Mojitos are a delicious cocktail created from lime, mint, and rum. The cocktail-inspired popsicle recipe includes rum, making it ideal for those seeking a refreshing treat on a hot summer day.

1½ cup water

1/2 cup freshly squeezed lime juice.

Ingredients: ½ cup sugar, ¼ cup fresh mint leaves, ¼ cup mild rum.

1. In a blender or food processor, combine water, lime juice, sugar, mint, and rum. Process until smooth and sugar dissolves completely. To remove mint leaves, strain through a fine strainer.

2. Pour into popsicle molds and freeze for 6 hours or overnight until solid.

Makes 6–8 popsicles.

Root Beer Float Pops

A root beer float is excellent with melted ice cream to add smoothness to the peppery soda. This pop is a delicious combination of sweet, spicy, and creamy Flavors.

12 ounces of root beer.

1/2 cup coconut milk.

1 teaspoon vanilla extract.

1. Mix root beer, coconut milk, and vanilla in a large basin. Refrigerate for 30 minutes to allow carbonation to dissipate.
2. Pour into popsicle molds and freeze for 6 hours or overnight until solid.
Makes 6–8 popsicles.

Coconut and Orange Creamsicles

Orange juice and vanilla make a delicious frozen pop. This dairy-free creamsicle combines fresh orange juice and coconut milk with a hint of vanilla. For a stronger orange flavor, use concentrated orange juice instead of store-bought juice.

1 cup of freshly squeezed orange juice.

1 tablespoon of Cointreau or other orange liqueur.

⅓ Cup Sugar

1 cup coconut milk.

¼ teaspoon vanilla extract.

1. In a large bowl, combine orange juice, Cointreau, and sugar. Whisk rapidly until sugar dissolves. Mix in coconut milk and vanilla.

2. Pour into popsicle molds and freeze for 6 hours or overnight until solid.

Makes 6–8 popsicles.

Avocado & Lime Creamsicles

Avocados are naturally creamy and heavy in fat.

While commonly associated with savory foods, they can also be combined with sugar and served as a dessert in some countries. This recipe creates a creamy, green popsicle that may convince you to try avocados for dessert.

Two ripe, medium Hass avocados

Add ½ cup water and ¼ cup freshly squeezed lime juice.

½ cup sugar

1. Blend or process avocados, water, lime juice, and sugar until smooth and sugar is completely dissolved.

2. Pour into popsicle molds and freeze for 6 hours or

overnight until solid.

Makes 6–8 popsicles.

Ice cream, while delicious on its own, can be enhanced with additional toppings. These recipes transform your favorite Flavors into delectable treats, like ice cream sandwiches and bonbons.

Double chocolate chip cookies

These cookies have a generous amount of cocoa powder and chocolate chips, making them the perfect indulgence. These cookies spread considerably during baking, making them ideal for making ice cream sandwiches. They can hold a lot of ice cream and still be bite-sized.

2 cups all-purpose flour.

1/2 teaspoon baking soda.

1 teaspoon salt.

1/2 cup shortening, vegan margarine, or coconut oil.

3/4 cup cocoa powder.

2 cups sugar.

1 teaspoon of vanilla extract.

⅔ cup soy milk

2 teaspoons of vinegar.

2 cups chocolate chips.

1. Preheat the oven to 350° Fahrenheit. Line a baking sheet with parchment paper.

2. Mix flour, baking soda, and salt in a medium bowl.

3. Melt the shortening in a small microwave-safe bowl.

4. In a large mixing bowl, combine melted shortening and cocoa powder. Whisk until smooth. Whisk in sugar, vanilla, soy milk, and vinegar. Gradually add the flour mixture and whisk until no flour streaks remain. Stir in the chocolate chips.

5. Place 1-inch dough balls on the prepared baking sheet, leaving about 2 inches between cookies to allow for spreading.

6. Bake cookies for 10-12 minutes, or until edges are firm.

7. Allow to cool on the baking sheet for 2-3 minutes before transferring to a wire rack to finish cooling.

Makes approximately 36 cookies.

Maple Chocolate Chip Cookies.

Chocolate chip cookies are a timeless classic. These cookies are versatile and can be enjoyed with milk, coffee, or as ice cream sandwiches. They are slightly crisp on the edges and delicate inside.

2 cups all-purpose flour.

1½ tsp baking powder.

1/2 teaspoon baking soda.

1 teaspoon salt.

½ cup sugar

1/2 cup vegetable oil.

⅔ cup maple syrup.

1 teaspoon of vanilla extract.

⅔ cup chocolate chips.

1. Preheat the oven to 350° Fahrenheit. Line a baking sheet with parchment paper.

2. Mix flour, baking powder, baking soda, salt, and sugar in a large bowl.

3. In a small bowl, whisk together the oil, maple syrup, and

vanilla.

Pour into the flour mixture, stirring until almost incorporated. Add chocolate chips and mix until there are no flour streaks.

Ice cream sandwiches and other frozen treats.

4. Roll into 1-inch spherical balls and set on baking sheet, leaving about 2 inches between cookies to allow for spreading.

5. Bake for 10-12 minutes until cookies are baked and hard around the edges. Allow to cool on the baking sheet for 2-3 minutes before transferring to a wire rack to cool fully.

Makes approximately 20 cookies.

Chewy Gingersnap Cookies

Chewy cookies are ideal for ice cream sandwiches as they maintain their texture better in the freezer than crunchy cookies, which can become rigid and difficult to bite into. These cookies are ideal for the end-of-year celebrations but also taste excellent year-round, especially when filled with ice cream.

2 cups all-purpose flour.

2 tablespoons cornstarch.

2 tablespoons baking soda.

¼ teaspoon salt

2 tbsp. ground ginger

1 teaspoon ground cinnamon.

¼ teaspoon ground cloves

1/4 teaspoon ground black pepper

1 cup sugar.

⅔ cup vegetable oil

⅓ cup molasses

1½ teaspoons orange juice.

1 tablespoon of orange zest.

1 teaspoon of vanilla extract.

⅔ cup sugar (for rolling)

1. Preheat the oven to 350° Fahrenheit. Line a baking sheet with parchment paper.

2. Mix flour, cornstarch, baking soda, salt, ginger, cinnamon, cloves, and pepper in a large basin.

Ice cream sandwiches and other frozen treats. 79

3. Combine sugar, oil, molasses, orange juice, zest, and

vanilla in a medium basin. Pour into the flour mixture and whisk until no dry components remain visible.

4. Roll dough into 1-inch balls, coat with sugar, and set on prepared baking sheet. Allow approximately 2 inches between cookies to spread.

5. Bake for 7–9 minutes until the edges of the cookies are firm. Don't overbake.

6. Allow cookies to cool for 3 to 5 minutes on the baking sheet before transferring to a wire rack to cool completely. Makes approximately 36 cookies.

Cream Bonbons

Ice cream bonbons are a frozen dessert with the same level of indulgence as truffles. Ice cream balls are dipped in molten chocolate to form a silky candy shell.

While you can use any flavour of ice cream, chocolate and vanilla are timeless Favorites. These can be stored in the freezer for several weeks if concealed below frozen peas; however, they are often consumed fast.

1⅓ cups ice cream of choice.

8 ounces of dark or semisweet chocolate

2 tablespoons coconut oil.

1. Make 12 ice cream balls with a diameter slightly smaller than 1 inch. Place ice cream balls on a parchment-lined baking sheet and freeze for 30-60 minutes.
Ice cream sandwiches and other frozen treats.

2. In a medium microwave-safe bowl, combine chocolate and coconut oil. Microwave for 30- to 40-second intervals, stirring with a spatula, until chocolate is melted and smooth. Allow to cool slightly.

3. Dip frozen ice cream balls into melted chocolate with two forks, then return to the baking sheet prepared with parchment paper. If the chocolate mixture thickens while working, reheat and stir. Repeat to coat all ice cream balls and freeze. This makes twelve bonbons.

Chocolate Affogato.

Affogato is an Italian dish that combines ice cream with coffee or espresso to create a "drowned" effect. A simple and elegant after-dinner drink, especially with a scoop of chocolate ice cream or sorbet that complements strong coffee.

1 scoop chocolate ice cream or bittersweet chocolate sorbet.

2 ounces of hot espresso or strong coffee

Place a scoop of ice cream in a small cup or dessert bowl.

Pour hot espresso on top and serve immediately. Serves 1

Adding a luscious topping to a dish of ice cream is a delightful way to enhance the experience.

Create your own sundae by combining your Favorite ice cream and topping varieties.

Quick-Setting Chocolate Sauce

Pour this simple chocolate sauce over ice cream to create a thin layer that can be cracked with a spoon. It sets quickly. It enhances the flavour and texture of your Favorite ice cream.

6 ounces of semisweet or dark chocolate, finely chopped

2½ teaspoons coconut oil.

1. In a medium microwave-safe bowl, combine chocolate and coconut oil. Microwave for 30- to 40-second intervals, stirring with a spatula, until chocolate is melted and smooth.

2. Drizzle or pour the sauce over the ice cream, then serve. Refrigerate leftovers in an airtight container and reheat them as needed.

This makes approximately 1 cup

Dark Chocolate Fudge Sauce

This chocolate sauce is full of flavour and ideal for chocolate lovers. This recipe combines cocoa powder and dark chocolate and pairs well with ice cream and cake. It can be added to hot chocolate or dipped in fruit!

1/2 cup cocoa powder.

Combine ¾ cup sugar and ¾ cup boiling water.

1 teaspoon of vanilla extract.

4 oz. dark chocolate, finely chopped

1. In a small saucepan, mix together cocoa powder, sugar, and boiling water until combined. Bring to a simmer over medium heat, stirring until sugar is dissolved and smooth.

2. Remove from heat, then add vanilla essence and dark chocolate. Stir until well integrated.

3. Drizzle or pour the sauce over the ice cream, then serve. Refrigerate leftovers in an airtight container and reheat them as needed.

Makes approximately 1 cup.

A delicious raspberry sauce pairs well with creamy ice cream. This sauce is simple to make and may be prepared on the stovetop or in the microwave. I prefer frozen berries because they are readily available, but fresh berries are also suitable.

1 cup of frozen raspberries.

1/4 cup strawberry or raspberry jam.

2 teaspoons sugar.

1 teaspoon of lemon juice.

1. Mix raspberries, jam, sugar, and lemon juice in a medium microwave-safe bowl. boil on high for 1 minute, then whisk and boil for another 60-90 seconds, until the syrup is bubbling and somewhat thick. (Alternatively, simmer raspberries, jam, sugar, and lemon juice in a small saucepan over medium heat, stirring frequently, until the mixture thickens.)

2. Let the mixture cool before covering and serving. Store

leftovers in an airtight jar in the fridge.

This makes approximately 1 cup

Vegan salted caramel sauce

Salted caramel is highly seductive due to its perfect balance of salt and sweetness. This sauce is ideal for topping an ice cream sandwich. To enhance the caramel flavour, boil the syrup until dark brown before adding the coconut milk. Use full-fat coconut milk for optimal results.

⅓ Cup water

1 cup sugar.

¾ cup coconut milk

1 teaspoon salt. 1 teaspoon of vanilla extract.

1. In a medium saucepan, heat water and sugar over medium heat. Stir with a spatula until sugar dissolves. Boil the syrup for 3 to 5 minutes, until it reaches a rich amber colour.

Sauces and toppings (87)

2. Combine the coconut milk with the hot caramel. The mixture will bubble vigorously. Stir in salt and vanilla until the sauce is smooth. Remove from heat and store in a

separate container.

3. Let the caramel sauce cool before covering and serving. Refrigerate leftovers in an airtight container and reheat them as needed. Makes approximately 1½ cups.

Coconut Cream Whipped Cream

This vegan whipped cream recipe uses coconut cream to create a light and fluffy texture. To achieve the best results, chill the coconut cream thoroughly before beginning. Keeping a can in the refrigerator ensures you always have some on hand.

1 can (15 ounces) coconut cream, chilled

3 tablespoons of confectioners' sugar.

1/2 teaspoon of vanilla extract (optional)

1. Pour the coconut cream into a large mixing basin. To make soft peaks, beat cream by hand or with an electric mixer at medium speed for 3 to 5 minutes.

2. Add confectioners' sugar, adjust to taste, and beat in. If using, add vanilla extract and beat briefly. Serve immediately.

Makes approximately 2 cups.

www.ingramcontent.com/pod-product-compliance
Lightning Source LLC
Chambersburg PA
CBHW050815250726